Knee Pain

Treating Knee Pain
Preventing Knee Pain
Natural Remedies, Medical Solutions, Along With Exercises And Rehab For Knee Pain Relief

By Ace McCloud
Copyright © 2014

Disclaimer

The information provided in this book is designed to provide helpful information on the subjects discussed. This book is not meant to be used, nor should it be used, to diagnose or treat any medical condition. For diagnosis or treatment of any medical problem, consult your own physician. The publisher and author are not responsible for any specific health or allergy needs that may require medical supervision and are not liable for any damages or negative consequences from any treatment, action, application or preparation, to any person reading or following the information in this book. Any references included are provided for informational purposes only. Readers should be aware that any websites or links listed in this book may change.

Table of Contents

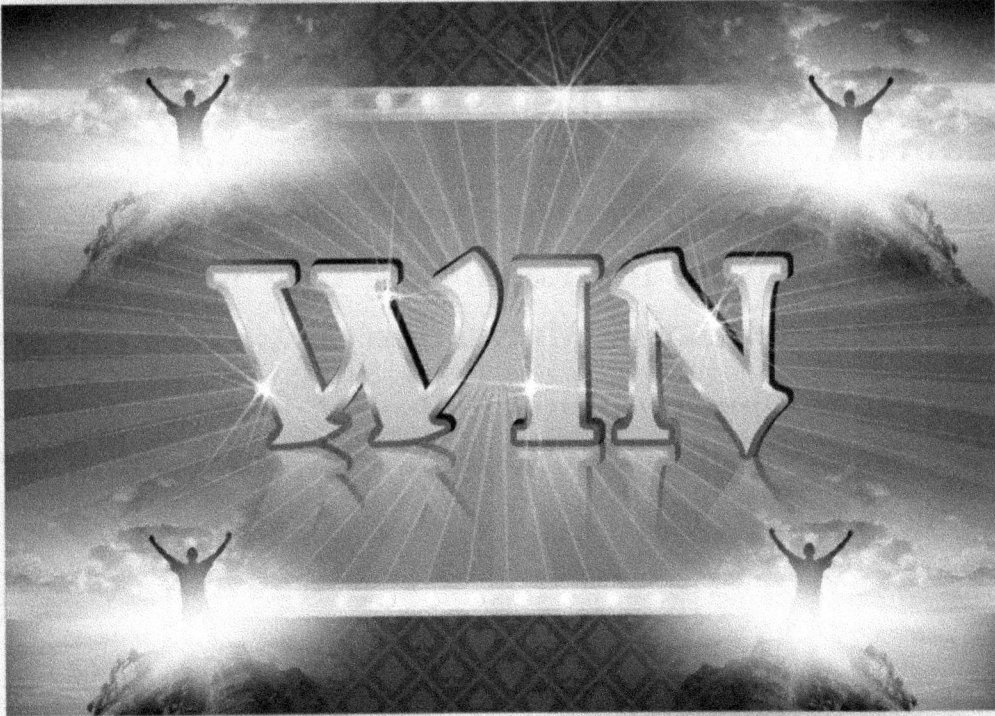

DEDICATED TO THOSE WHO ARE PLAYING THE GAME OF LIFE TO

WIN

KEEP ON PUSHING AND NEVER GIVE UP!

Ace McCloud

Be sure to check out my website for all my Books and Audio books.

www.AcesEbooks.com

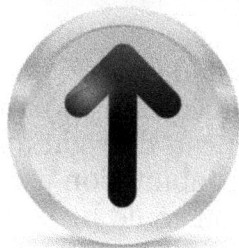

Introduction

I want to thank you and congratulate you for buying the book, "Knee Pain Cure: How To Treat Knee Pain, How To Prevent Knee Pain, All Natural Remedies For Knee Pain, Medical Cures For Knee Pain, Along With Exercises And Rehab For Knee Pain Relief."

This book contains proven steps and strategies on how to prevent knee pain and how to treat it using the best medical and all natural methods. Learn basic knee-strengthening exercises that you can do right at home and how to mentally get yourself through a knee injury rehabilitation process. There is no reason for you to suffer from knee pain when you could be taking steps to prevent it and make your knees stronger.

The information provided in this book is not meant to be a substitute for professional medical advice or treatment. Always consult a professional doctor when it comes to your health.

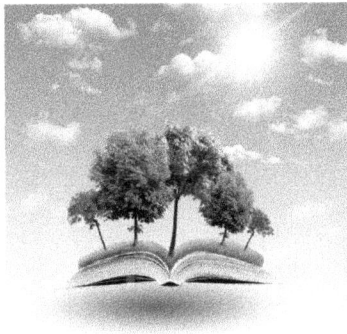

Chapter 1: What Causes Knee Pain?

Our knees are one of the most important parts of our body because they serve as our support system. Our knees enable us to bend, straighten, stand, walk, run, jump, and perform any other similar motion. Unfortunately, body parts are prone to accidents and medical problems. Knee problems are not discriminating: they occur in men, women, and children of all backgrounds. The most common causes of knee pain and injuries are in impact sports, falling or direct impact accidents, and overuse of the knees in general. Our bones, cartilage, muscles, ligaments, and tendons all help our knees function correctly. If any of these parts are hurt or worn out, our knees are at risk of being unable to function correctly.

There are two categories of knee injuries: medical and inflammatory. Medical-related knee injuries are a result of a direct impact or a sudden, wrong movement. Inflammatory-related injuries are a result of certain diseases that cause swelling, such as arthritis. Whether you are an athlete or not, knee pain can affect almost anyone.

A doctor can diagnose a medical or inflammatory-related knee injury through a physical examination and by performing a series of diagnostic tests such as a CAT scan or MRI. Orthopaedists are the best types of doctors to consult because they specialize in bone, cartilage, ligament, and tendon problems. Below is a list of the most common causes of knee pain.

Arthritis

Arthritis is one condition that is commonly connected to knee pain, especially when you put continuous wear and tear on your knees. Osteoarthritis is a form of arthritis that affects the knees by causing the cartilage to erode. Another type of arthritis that commonly affects the knees is rheumatoid arthritis. Rheumatoid arthritis inflames the cartilage around the knees and essentially destroys it.

Cartilage Injuries

Cartilage injuries are another common cause of knee pain. A condition called Chondromalacia occurs when the knee cap cartilage gets soft and easily tears. This can occur due to an injury, excessive use, or a weakening of the muscles. One piece of cartilage that is susceptible to injury is the meniscus, which is a c-shaped piece of cartilage that pads the area between your thigh bone and shin bone. If your knee gets twisted under a lot of weight, the cartilage in this area can tear. Depending on the circumstances, the tear can either be small or large. Small cartilage injuries can last up to six weeks. Large cartilage injuries may require surgery.

Ligament Injuries

Ligament injuries are often called sprains. These types of injuries commonly occur during aggressive contact sports such as football or hockey. The two most commonly injured ligaments include the anterior cruciate ligament (ACL) and the posterior cruciate ligament (PCL). Injuries to the ACL are usually the results of over-stretching or a sudden movement. Injuries to the PCL are usually the results of a direct blow. A direct impact to the outer side of the knees can cause damage to the medial and lateral collateral ligaments. The time it takes for a ligament injury to heal depends on the severity and location of the the injury. In the case of a sprain or small tear to the outer knee, healing usually takes up to three months. If the tear is bigger it can take up to 9 months. If you require surgery for injuries related to the ACL or PCL, healing can take six to twelve months.

Tendon Injuries

The three primary types of tendon injuries are tendinitis, Osgood-Schlatter disease, and iliotibal band syndrome. Playing sports that require jumping, such as basketball, sometimes cause tendinitis (also known as 'jumper's knee'). Too much jumping can cause the tendons to become inflamed. Ruptured tendons occur from overuse and when your thigh muscles contract (like if you are trying to break a fall). Stress and tension on the upper shin bone can cause Osgood-Schlatter disease, which causes swelling when the tendon tears away from the bone. Osgood-Schlatter disease often occurs in younger people. When a tendon rubs over the outer bone of the knee over a long period of time, it can cause swelling known as iliotibal band syndrome. A mildly inflamed tendon can take only a few weeks to heal. A badly inflamed tendon can take up to a few months to heal.

Osteochondritis Dissecans

Osteochondritis dissecans occurs when too little blood flows to the bone under a joint surface. This causes the bone and cartilage to loosen and become painful. Some of the cartilage may even break off and cause the joints to lock in a sharp pain. If osteochondritis dissecans occurs and is not treated it can develop into osteoarthritis. Sometimes, osteochondritis dissecans requires operative surgery to prevent it from developing into osteoarthritis.

These are the main causes of knee injuries and knee pain. They are all different and can affect almost anyone, depending on their age and their activities. The rest of this book will cover the topics of how to prevent these pains and injuries, how to use both medical and natural methods to ease the pains, how to exercise your knees as method of rehabilitation and strength-building, and how to mentally prepare yourself to undergo the rehabilitation process.

Chapter 2: How to Prevent Knee Pain

Knee pain is some of the worst pain you may ever experience, especially since your knees serve as the support system for your body. Luckily, there are some proven methods that you can take advantage of to help to try and prevent yourself from suffering knee pain. Stretching and strength-training will help you reduce your likelihood of experiencing a painful knee-injury. If you're suffering from knee pain, protective braces or wraps can help soothe the pain.

Stretching

Since our muscles need oxygen-rich blood to work properly, we should always stretch before and after physical activity. Not only does stretching feel good, but it allows more blood to flow through our circulatory system, which helps our muscles when we move. Stretching also helps us become more flexible, stronger, and have better circulation. If you focus and stretch in a quiet area you can also even bring down your levels of stress.

The best way to stretch is to hold yourself in a stretching position for 30 to 60 seconds. This gives your muscles a chance to warm up and become flexible. Never stretch beyond a way that is uncomfortable to you and never rush. Most doctors recommend that you stretch for 10 minutes before physical activity and 10 minutes after.

Strength-Training

There are many studies that support the idea that strength training helps prevent injuries of all kinds but specifically knee injuries, in this case. Strength training allows your bones to get used to physical activity, which may decrease your chance of experiencing bone deterioration. Strength training also has a positive effect on your ligaments and tendons because it will increase their size and strength, making them more resistant to injury. Finally, strength training has a positive effect on your muscles. The lower your muscle strength, the higher your chances are of falling and fracturing your knees. Persistent strength-training will significantly lower your chances of getting injured.

Protective Braces or Wraps

Protective knee braces or wraps are another way to protect yourself against knee injuries and the pain that follows. Health and fitness companies design these products to provide different levels of support and comfort to your knees. There are all sorts of braces and wraps available to help you. They are generally divided into four support categories: basic, advanced, elite, and knee pads.

Basic braces are elastic, cheap, and good for mild knee injuries. Advanced braces usually utilize Velcro straps and are good for moderate knee injuries. Elite braces provide advanced support and are best for severe knee injuries or post-surgery recovery. Here are some great knee braces: <u>Bracoo Neoprene Knee Support</u> and <u>Shock Doctor Knee Supporter</u>.

Finally, knee pads are made out of gel and provide comfort for people who are often on their knees. Gardeners and roofers, for example, would benefit from knee pads. The gel will help reduce the pressure you put on your knees, therefore causing less pain. Knee pads are good for those who suffer from Osgood-Schlatter disease and arthritis. Here are some great knee pads: <u>Fiskars Ultra Light Knee Pads</u>.

To protect yourself against knee pain or from incurring an injury in the future, be sure to stretch before and after you engage in physical activity, utilize strength-training to build up your muscles, and wear protective braces to keep your knees safe.

Chapter 3: The Best Medical Solutions for Preventing Knee Pain

When knee pain cannot be cured by methods such as over-the-counter medicines, ice packs, and rest, many people turn to knee surgery. Doctors will often first try non-surgical methods to cure knee pain before they recommend surgery. Since there are many causes of knee pain, there are many different types of surgeries that one can undergo to cure knee pain. Below is a list of the most common kinds of knee surgeries.

Meniscectomy

Doctors perform meniscectomy surgeries to remove a torn meniscus from the knee-joint. Many people suffering from knee pain undergo this surgery when a torn meniscus is causing them discomfort. During a meniscectomy surgery, a doctor will make a 1-centimeter incision and insert a small camera in the joint to aid them in the repair. He will then use small scissors to remove the torn meniscus. Afterward, the doctor will use the small camera to inspect the area and check for signs of arthritis and other potential joint problems. A meniscectomy surgery is generally painless. Often times, the patient will be put under an anesthetic before the surgery. Once the surgery is complete, it will only take patients a few days to return to their normal activities.

Meniscus Repair

If you tear your meniscus so badly that it prevents you from bending your knees, fully straightening your knees, or if you hear a popping sound when you do, your doctor might recommend a meniscus repair. However, this is only possible if the tear is around the outer edge of the knee, otherwise it will not heal. During a meniscus repair, your doctor will place tacks around or suture the torn edges. Both techniques allow the edges to heal in the right position. If your doctor removes the entire meniscus, you will be able to walk within a couple of days. However, if your doctor repairs your meniscus, post-rehabilitation is essential.

Meniscus Transplant

People who have their meniscus removed often undergo a meniscus transplant to further reduce knee pain. Some people prefer a meniscus transplant over a joint replacement. It is also an option when anti-inflammatory medicines do not work. Without a meniscus, your bone will gradually be exposed as the cartilage wears away. However, a meniscus transplant is not for everybody. The ideal candidate for a meniscus transplant is between 20-25 years old, has previously had his or her meniscus removed, has experienced limited damage to the bone lining of their joint, and displays symptoms consistent with having no meniscus. Once you have undergone a meniscus transplant, you will have to walk with crutches for four to six weeks although the entire healing process can take up to six months.

Lateral Release

A lateral release surgery helps doctors realign your kneecap. If your kneecap is pulled in a way where it ends up outside of its groove it can cause cartilage irritation and pain. Tight tissue on the outside of the kneecap often causes the pull. A doctor must assess your kneecap to determine if a lateral release surgery will work for you. In the past, doctors performed lateral release surgeries on many people, only to find out that it did not relieve their pain. In recent years, doctors and surgeons have gotten better at determining who will benefit from a lateral release.

Plica Excision

The inner side of your knee is most susceptible to injury and irritation. This area of the knee is known as the plica. Doctors prefer to treat plica syndrome with anti-inflammatory medicine but will perform surgery if medicine does not relieve the pain. During a plica excision, your doctor will insert a small camera into your knee and uses small instruments to remove the plica.

ACL Reconstruction

People who need a new ACL in their knee-joint undergo ACL reconstruction surgery. During the first phase of this surgery, your doctor will use a camera to determine the damage to your knee-joint as well as look for other damage. Once your doctor confirms a tear in your ACL, he or she must obtain a graft.

The three most common types of ACL grafts are patellar tendon grafts, hamstring tendon grafts, and donor grafts. Once the doctor has obtained the graft, he or she prepares the tissue to fit the new ACL. Next, your doctor will drill a hole to create a tunnel in the shin bone to make a place for the new ACL. Once this is done, your doctor will pass your new ACL through the tunnel using a large pin. Then the doctor will fix the graft in place by screwing it into the end of the tunnel.

Quadriceps Tendon Repair

Our quadriceps tendon is just above our knee cap and is what allows us to bend our knees or kick. The quadriceps muscle, the quad tendon, the knee cap, and the pateller make up the quadriceps tendon. Though our quadriceps tendon is a strong muscle, many people still get injuries by fracturing their kneecap, tearing their pateller tendon, or tearing their quad tendon. Many doctors misdiagnose a slightly torn quad tendon as a kneecap issue. A slightly torn quad tendon does not require surgery, however, a completely torn quad tendon does. If you have a completely torn quad tendon you won't be able to straighten your leg. Your doctor should perform surgery within a couple of weeks of the injury to ensure a full recovery. During the surgical procedure, your doctor will suture the torn tendon back to the kneecap by drilling holes in the bone and pulling the tendon through them. Afterward, you will wear a brace, use crutches, and undergo physical therapy for three months.

Knee Replacement Surgery

If you are suffering from a severe case of arthritis you might consider undergoing a full knee replacement surgery. Many people consider this option when non-surgical treatments have failed. If you choose to undergo a full knee replacement surgery, your doctor will give you an anesthetic and then remove all the bone and cartilage that is between your thigh and shin bone through a large incision. Once your doctor has removed everything, he or she will work on putting an implant in you. Your doctor will either cement the implant to your bone or use the "press-fit" method, which allows your bone to grow into the implant. The entire surgery takes between 60 and 90 minutes. Afterward, your doctor will most likely recommend rehabilitation to help you get used to your new knee.

Partial Knee Replacement

Many people consider a Partial knee replacement as a non-invasive surgery. One of the most common reasons for a partial knee replacement is a very bad case of arthritis in the knee. Partial knee replacement has a relatively short recovery time and only requires a small incision. The main goal of the surgery is to remove badly damaged cartilage and replace it with implants. Doctors only recommend a partial knee replacement for those who are older than 55 years of age with a healthy weight and whose ligaments are still intact. If you wait too long to have this type of surgery, the arthritis may become too advanced and severely decrease the success rate of the surgery.

Same-Day Knee Replacement

Same-day knee replacement surgery is like traditional knee placement surgery except that it is minimally invasive. Since your doctor does not need to cut your quadriceps tendon during the procedure, you will benefit from a fast recovery time, less medication, and a shorter duration of physical therapy. A same-day knee replacement surgery only requires a 3 to 4-inch incision and uses the same implants as a traditional knee replacement surgery. Like its name, same-day knee placement allows you to go home on the same day of the surgery because rehab starts before you even leave the hospital. Same day knee surgery is usually recommended for those with no diabetes or heart problems around the ages of fifty four to sixty six years of age.

Cold Laser Therapy

Cold laser therapy is a relatively new technique that relieves knee pain without the need for surgery. Doctors have used cold laser therapy to relieve meniscus tears, arthritis pains, tendinitis, failed surgery, and other causes of knee pain. Cold laser therapy is a popular option because it is painless and non-invasive. During the treatment, your doctor will use a device that sends wavelengths of light to the area of pain. The light from the laser reaches into the tissue of your body and helps stimulate damaged cells, which helps increase their rate of healing. It also reduces inflammation. Cold laser therapy has also proven to improve tissue and cell health. In mild cases of knee pain, cold laser therapy can almost immediately relieve your pain. However, depending on the length and severity of your pain or injury, it takes about an average of 10 to 30 treatments to feel relief.

Makoplasty

Makoplasty is a new, alternative type of knee replacement method that a computer and robot guides. Makoplasty stands out from a human-guided surgery because a robot is much more precise and accurate. During a makoplasty procedure, your doctor will use a 3D CAT scan to guide a robotic arm in preserving your healthy bone and tissue while resurfacing the damaged parts. Makoplasty is minimally invasive and has a quicker recovery time than if it were human-guided.

Human Growth Hormone

A human growth hormone is a chemical copy of the natural growth hormones that our bodies create. Doctors generally administer doses of human growth hormone by an injection. Studies have shown that human growth hormone injections can increase protein production in knee-joints and muscles. The studies also suggest that human growth hormone injections can promote the healing of knee injuries and muscle injuries.

There are many medical solutions to knee injuries and knee pains. Depending on your injury, you may best benefit from human-guided surgery, a laser treatment, a robot-guided surgery, or even from a medical substance such as human growth hormone. Many people turn to these methods when regular rest and over-the-counter medicines like ibuprofen do not work. However, some people like to try all natural methods before turning to medical methods. Some of the best all-natural approaches against knee pain may get the job done without the need for surgery.

Chapter 4: All Natural Approaches For Knee Pain

All-natural approaches for knee pain are popular because they are less expensive than medical solutions and do not require a trip to a doctor's office or hospital. The nice thing about the all-natural approach is that they are usually less costly and a lot safer than some of the medical alternatives. They can also be done in the comfort of your own home, a nice bonus.

PRICE

PRICE is an acronym for "protect, rest, ice, compression, and elevation." It represents the most basic, natural, and time-tested knee injury healing method. Following the PRICE method is a great rule of thumb for whenever you incur a knee injury. I have used this method personally with great success on several occasions.

If you sustain a knee injury, you should "protect" your soft tissue by wrapping your knee with a bandage, brace, or wrap. Protecting it will shorten your recovery time and can prevent the injury from getting worse.

Next, you should "rest" your injury to avoid continuously straining it. Resting it also helps shorten your recovery time and ensures that the injury will heal right. The most important time to rest your injury is right after it happens and then for the next couple of days. However, it is important to move it after a few days so that your muscles don't grow weak.

In addition to resting your injury right away, you should also "ice" it immediately. Applying ice on your injury for 10-15 minutes can greatly reduce swelling. You can apply ice to your injury by using an instant ice pack, an ice bag, or a cold knee wrap. "Compression" can also be applied during the icing step. For example, a cold knee wrap will ice and compress your injury at the same time. Compression also helps prevent swelling. A great knee wrap is: Brownmed Polar Ice Knee Wrap.

Finally, "elevation" also reduces swelling by draining excess fluid out of the injured area. The best way to elevate your knee is to lie down on your back and support your leg with pillows. There is no special time limit on how long you should elevate your knee—it is up to you to determine when you feel better.

PRICE is a great method to follow, especially during the first few days of a knee injury. To be precautionary, you should always follow up with a doctor, but until you can make a doctor's appointment, PRICE can help you manage your injury and feel comfortable.

Natural Healing Supplements

Many people prefer to heal their knee injuries and knee pains with natural and homeopathic remedies before turning to medical solutions. Many natural and homeopathic solutions are best suited for treating osteoarthritis, although most of them reduce the inflaming and pain that injuries can cause. Researchers have conducted studies on many of these solutions and have discovered that they work. Remember that natural and herbal methods are not usually tested for side effects and you should consult with your doctor before trying any of the products listed below.

Omega-3 Fatty Acids

Omega-3 fatty acids are a common, natural remedy used to treat knee pain in those who suffer from arthritis. Originally found in fish, many doctors believe that omega-3 fatty acids reduce inflammation. Studies show that omega-3 fatty acids reduced pain and tiredness in those who suffer from rheumatoid arthritis. You can increase your intake of omega-3 fatty acids by buying supplements or you can eat foods that contain it, such as fish or flaxseed. Always check with your doctor before taking an omega-3 fatty acid supplement because some of them can contain toxic levels of mercury or Vitamin A. My favorite omega 3 fatty acid is: Nature Made Fish Oil Omega-3.

Glucosamine

Glucosamine is a natural substance that is in your joints and connective tissue. It helps repair cartilage and keeps your joints flexible. Glucosamine supplements may also slow down cartilage deterioration. There have been a variety of reports that shows glucosamine has been found to help those who suffer from arthritis-related knee pain. You can choose from two types of glucosamine: glucosamine sulfate and glucosamine hydrochloride. Many people prefer to take 1,500 mg of glucosamine sulfate per day. My favorite glucosamine product is: Schiff Glucosamine plus MSM.

Chondroitin

Chondroitin is best for minimizing pain, improving joints, and fending off arthritis. Many people prefer to take chondroitin supplements because it does not cause any major side effects, although it can take up to a month to notice any changes in your body.

Glucosamine+Chondroitin

Instead of taking individual doses of glucosamine and chondroitin, many people take a combined supplement. Together, they work as a powerful painkiller. The National Institute of Health found that a combination of glucosamine and chondroitin work best to relieve pain in those who suffer from mild to moderate knee pain. Those who suffer from moderate to severe pain are better off taking individual doses, as the study did not show any significant pain relief in that group.

I recommend the Doctor's Best brand of this combination pill, which can be found here : Doctor's Best – Glucosmaine/Chondroitin/MSM.

Each bottle comes with 240 capsules and sells for an average of a little under $25. Doctor's Best Glucosamine/Chondroitin MSM helped me reduce the amount of pain that my workout routine was putting on my knees. After taking two capsules a day for 7 days, I felt as if my pain was never there in the first place.

Sam-E

Sam-E is a natural knee pain remedy that stimulates blood flow. Studies have proven that Sam-E is comparable to other anti-inflammatory medicines except that it does not have any major side effects.

Avocado Soybean Unsaponifiables

Avocados and soybeans make up a homeopathic knee pain treatment that can prevent cartilage erosion and promote healing. It also protects your knees against arthritis and reduces inflammation. A great product that has Glucosamine, Chondroitin, Avocado and Soybeans is: Cosamin ASU Active People.

Boswellia

Boswellia is another word for Indian Frankincense. Medical studies show that it can decrease arthritis pain in some people by up to 80%. A good Boswellia supplement is: Nature's Way Boswellia.

Ginger

Ginger is a great natural remedy for joint problems. Ginger can increase your blood circulation and block chemicals from affecting your joints. One medical study shows that 75% of people who take one dose of ginger per day reported feeling relief from their arthritis pains. Nature's Made Ginger is a great product you may want to check out.

Evening Primrose Oil

Evening primrose oil is a fatty acid that can help people with rheumatoid arthritis. It also helps reduce knee pain and stiffness. However, evening primrose oil is only effective with taken by mouth. Nature's Way EFA Gold Evening Primrose is a good supplement you may want to try.

Proper Diet=Quicker Recovery

Eating a proper diet can help you keep your bones strong and will decrease your chance of sustaining a knee injury. Certain foods can help strengthen your bones and joints and prevent fractures, deterioration, and muscle growth.

Protein, which you can get from foods such as red meats, can make your bones stronger by helping increase their mineral content. Protein can also build muscle and encourage muscle growth during strength-training activities. Many doctors recommend that you get protein from eggs, salmon, red meats, soy, beans, and legumes. My favorite protein supplement of all time is: Muscle Milk.

While protein can help promote bone mineral content, refined sugars have an opposite effect and you should cut them out of your diet to protect your bones. In particular, carbonated soft drinks and even sports drinks like Gatorade (which is commonly targeted to athletes) can cause a decrease in bone minerals. Refined sugars can also lead to a number of other bone problems such as a decrease in muscle mass. Many doctors recommend that you should choose beverages such as milk or juice over sodas due to their nutritious vitamin content.

Speaking of milk, many doctors recommend a diet that is rich in calcium and vitamin D to help protect yourself from bone deterioration or injuries. Calcium is a major player in our bodies and is even more important for our bones because it helps them grow stronger. You can get your daily intake of calcium by drinking milk or calcium-fortified juice or through dairy products such as cheese or yogurt. Vitamin D helps your bones absorb calcium so it is important for you to make sure that you are getting enough of this vitamin as well. Our bodies produce vitamin D when it is exposed to sunlight and it is also found in foods such as fish, egg yolks, orange juice, and cow's milk. If you think your diet may be lacking in Calcium or Vitamin D, here is a good supplement that provides both nutrients: Vitafusion Calcium with Vitamin D Gummy Vitamins.

Finally, carbohydrates play an important role in bone health. Complex carbohydrates, which are found in fruits and vegetables, help your bones absorb calcium and can increase your bone mass density.

Overall, a proper diet will not only protect your bones but it will protect your overall health. It will keep you energized, feeling good, and healthy. One final option to making sure that you are getting enough vitamins and minerals is to take supplements, such as multivitamins. However, by simply maintaining a healthy diet, you can help your bones to grow strong and lower your chances of sustaining a bad injury from weak bones. If you would like more information on healthy living, be sure to check out my book: Anti-Aging Cure.

Light Therapy

Light therapy is the method of using infrared and LED light to relieve pain by relaxing your muscle tissue. Many people suffering from knee pain look into light therapy because it is an alternative to using drugs or medicine. NASA originally discovered the benefits of using infrared lights for therapy during plant growth experiments.

During a light therapy process, those who are suffering from knee pain expose their knee to a set of infrared and LED lights for a short time period (usually 17-20 minutes) twice a day. Devices that are specifically designed for knees often come with Velcro straps so that you can strap it right on to your knee. Since everyone's pain and injuries are different, the time it takes to heal and feel better will depend from person to person. However, light therapy is proven to work on all skin types and is safe and painless.

Clinical studies have shown that light therapy can speed up the healing process of an injury by boosting circulation and blocking chemicals that cause pain sensations. It also increases the amount of endorphins that your body produces and can help relieve swelling. Finally, it stimulates the synthesis of RNA and DNA, which can replace damaged cells. A great product that makes use of light therapy is TenDLite Red LED Light Therapy.

Heat Therapy

Heat therapy for knee pain is best used for chronic conditions. Heat therapy relaxes your muscles, stimulates your circulation, and loosens your tissues. You can engage in a simple heat therapy method by simply using a towel soaked in hot water or by using a heating pad. You should never use a heat therapy method for more than 20 minutes at a time or to treat a mild injury.

Cold Therapy

Cold therapy can relieve pain, swelling, and inflammation caused by knee pain. The most common cold therapy treatment is a simple ice bag. You can fill a bag with ice and apply it to your knee.

Another common cold therapy method is an ice compression pack. An ice compression pack can easily wrap around your leg while providing a stable source of coldness.

One of the best ice compression packs I have used in the past is the Brownmed Polar Ice Knee Wrap.

I particularly like this ice wrap because it's soft, flexible, and it is easy to use. Although it only stays cold for about 30 minutes, the removable ice packs are small so they re-freeze quickly. I would highly recommend this product to anyone who wants to use cold therapy for knee pain.

Finally, instant ice packs are perfect for "emergency" situations because you do not have to wait for them to freeze at all. If you get injured and experience sudden knee pain, you can simply squeeze the pack and have instant access to ice for about 20 minutes. Instant ice packs are portable and can easily be stored in a basic first aid kit. Dynarex Instant Cold Pack is a good choice for instant ice.

The PRICE method as well as natural supplements, cold therapy, heat therapy, and light therapy are great, all natural ways to heal your knee injury at home, especially if they do not need medical attention. Once your injury heals, the next step that you will have to take is to bring your knee back up to strength.

Chapter 5: Exercising and Rehabbing Your Knees

Exercise is crucial for strengthening your knees, especially after an injury or surgery. If you have rested your knees after an injury or surgery and have not used them for a few days or weeks, you will need to exercise them to restore their strength and to rebuild muscle. Many orthopaedic surgeons recommend that you engage in 20 to 30 minutes of exercise twice a day until your knees are rehabbed. While some people may enter a physical therapy treatment program after a surgery, others practice an exercise regimen at home.

Basic Knee Exercises

Basic knee exercises are good for when you are just getting over an injury or a surgery. There are 15 basic strength-training knee exercises that you can engage in to help restore your knees. It is a good idea to start of gradually, and then work your way up to more intense exercises later on. You can turn many of these basic exercises into strength-training exercises by holding hand weights or attaching ankle weights to yourself.

Hamstring Contraction

You should do three sets of this exercise, around 10 reps each set. Sit on the floor or lie down and bend your knees at a 10 degree angle. Bring your heel to the floor and tighten your hamstring muscles, holding that position for five seconds.

Quadriceps Contraction

You should do three sets of this exercise, around 10 reps each set. Lie on your stomach and place a rolled towel under the ankle below your injured knee. Push your ankle into the towel while straightening your leg as much as you can while holding the position for five seconds.

Straight Leg Raises

You should do three sets of this exercise, around 10 reps each set. Start by Lying on your back with your healthy knee slightly bent while keeping your injured knee straight. Start by slowly lifting your injured knee six inches off of the ground. Hold this position for five seconds before lowering your knee back to the ground. A good example of this exercise can be seen on YouTube: Straight Leg Raises on YouTube.

Buttock Tucks

You should repeat this exercise 10 times with a total of three sets. For this exercise, simply lie on your back and tighten your buttock muscles for five seconds.

Standing Straight Leg Raises

You should do three sets of this exercise, around 10 reps each set. Support yourself using a wall or a banister and slowly lift your leg while keeping your knee straight. Hold the position for five seconds before bringing it back down.

Terminal Knee Extension

You should do three sets of this exercise, around 10 reps each set. Lie on your back and place a rolled towel under your bent knee. Straighten your knee and hold the position for seven seconds before relaxing. A great YouTube video of the Terminal Knee Extension by NoLimitAthlete can be seen here: TKE Terminal Knee Extension Video.

Straight Leg Raises (More Advanced)

You should perform 10-15 repetitions of this exercise for five full sets. Lie on your back with your good knee bent and straighten your injured knee using a quadriceps muscle contraction. Then, slowly raise your leg up to 12 inches off of the floor before bringing it back and relaxing.

Partial Chair Squat

You should repeat this exercise 10 times. Support yourself with a stable chair or a stable surface such as a counter. Place your feet 6 to 12 inches away from your support and squat with your back straight but do not go all the way down. Hold the position for 10 seconds and then go back up.

Standing Quadriceps Stretch

You should repeat this exercise 10 times with a total of three sets. While standing, bend your injured knee while slowly pulling your foot towards your buttocks. Continue to do this until you feel a good stretch. Hold this position for seven seconds and then relax. A great YouTube video by Livestrong.com of the standing quadriceps stretch can be seen here: How to Do the Standing Quad Stretch.

Knee Marching

You should repeat this exercise for one minute a day, twice a day. Sit in a chair and move your legs in a marching motion. This exercise can strengthen your knees and also prevent them from getting stiff while you're sitting for a long period of time.

Half Squats

You should repeat 3 sets of 10 of this exercise. Stand with your feet shoulder distance apart. Squat down about 12 inches and hold this position for ten seconds while placing the majority of your weight on your heels. Rise back up and then repeat after a short rest.

Leg Press

You should repeat 3 sets of 10 of this exercise. Using an elastic stretch band, lie on the floor and place the arc of your foot in the center of the band. Bring your bad knee toward your chest, hold the position for two seconds, and then slowly bring it back to its original position.

Walking

Walking is a great way to exercise and rehab your knees, especially after a knee replacement surgery. After a surgery, your doctor may give you a walker or pair of crutches to walk with as well as a limit on how much weight to put on your knees. However, walking on your own is the best way to heal your knees. Once you are able to walk without support, many doctors recommend that you continue to walk for at least 20 minutes a day to keep your knees strong. Walking is a safe, low-impact injury that can help rehab your knees.

When walking, be sure to stand upright and take short, small steps. Try not to overstep or step too far. Walking helps build muscle, bone density, and slows the loss of calcium from bones. Walking can even make you feel more energized. Overall, walking is a great, healthy activity that not only strengthens your knees but brings many positive benefits to your overall health.

When walking to heal a knee injury, it is important to make sure that you are wearing the right pair of shoes. A shoe without a good arch and level of comfort will only make matters worse. One way to ensure this without having to buy brand new shoes is to use gel inserts.

One product that I highly recommend is: RunPro Insoles. These inserts are great for keeping your foot in the right position to prevent injuries or stress on your knees. They are good for walking or for running.

Swimming

Swimming is another great way to exercise your knees because the water's buoyancy takes most of the stress of your body weight away. Swimming is a great way to work out and increase your overall health. By simply swimming regularly, your knees can grow strong because of the resistance that the water creates. You can also focus on exercising your knees by holding a kick-board while swimming laps. To exercise your quads and hamstrings, hold on to the side of the pool, face away from the wall, and sweep your leg back and forth at a 90-degree angle. Swimming exercises are also great for when you have arthritis in the knees.

Tips on Exercising

- Make sure you are wearing shoes with good support.
- Do not exercise on hard surfaces.
- Always warm up and stretch before engaging in exercise.
- Focus on the muscles that support your knees.
- Avoid exercises that require jumping.

Basic knee exercises, walking, and swimming are the top best ways to begin to move and rehabilitate your knees after sustaining an injury. Exercising your knees will also make them stronger so that they become more resistant to future injuries.

Chapter 6: Rehabilitation Motivation

After undergoing a knee surgery, you will most likely need to rehab your knee for it to work normally again. Experiencing a knee injury alone is hard because you have to watch others continue to go about their daily lives while your injury limits your abilities. After a surgery, some people may find the idea of rehabbing their knee as boring and tedious. Some people may even fall into a depression. However, the key to motivating yourself through a knee injury and physical therapy is to have a positive outlook. A positive outlook will help you maintain an upbeat attitude throughout the rehabilitation process and can even shorten the length of time it will take for your injury to heal. If you would like more information on maintaining a positive outlook and bringing more joy and laughter into your life, be sure to check out my bestselling book: Laughter Therapy.

The first crucial piece of advice for making it through your rehabilitation is to find the right physical therapist. Start this process before you even undergo surgery. Be sure to ask questions that can help you find a good match. Try to view your physical therapist as your main motivator. He or she is there to help you heal through encouragement and good advice. If you do not think that your physical therapist is a good match for you, do not be afraid to seek out a new one.

Music is also a great motivator. Most rehabilitation centers have music playing in the background but sometimes your physical therapist will allow you to bring your own music. Different music motivates different people so be sure to ask. You can also listen to music during your down time to keep your spirits up.

One way to mentally get through your rehabilitation process is to take advantage of your down time. You can use the extra time that you now have to review your goals, enhance your personal responsibility, and to mentally prepare yourself for getting into a rehab routine. You can also use your downtime to read up on your injury and learn more about it. Learning about your injury can help you keep track of its healing time and you can have engaging conversations about it with your physical therapist. It will also help you understand how the exercises in your routine are helping you heal. It is also a good idea to use visualization to see your knee as being totally healed and strong.

Another way to get through your rehabilitation process is to take advantage of your strong support system. Keep in touch with your friends and family members who are good at listening or see if you can talk to someone who has had a similar injury. If you don't have any friends or family members who had a similar injury, you can probably befriend somebody at the rehabilitation office. Your physical therapist may even be able to schedule you and your friend together, which can be very helpful in terms of support and motivation. By knowing that you have people who are supportive of you, you will be more inspired to go through with your rehabilitation. It will also feel good to know that you have people in your life who are willing to help you out in a time of need.

Finally, don't forget to talk to yourself—positively. You might find yourself thinking negative thoughts such as, "my sports career is over," or "I will never walk the same again." Instead of thinking those thoughts, set goals for yourself and think about achieving them. You will find yourself working hard to reach those goals and feeling great about your injury and yourself.

Rehabilitating your knee can be challenging. However, don't let that challenge be one that you fail. If you are an athlete, treat the challenge of physical therapy the same way that you would treat a sports game. If you are not an athlete, try to compare your goal to another goal that you would usually be working toward. By making sure that you have a good physical therapist, are taking advantage of your down time, have a strong support system, and are thinking positively, you can make your rehabilitation process more uplifting than depressing. If all goes well, your knee will be stronger than ever in no time!

Conclusion

I hope this book was able to help you to learn how to prevent and heal knee pain by using medicine, all natural methods, as well as exercises and supplements.

The next step is to make a rehab plan and follow through with it. Be sure you are doing everything consistently and that you are not doing so much that you re-injure your knee.

Finally, if you discovered at least one thing that has helped you or that you think would be beneficial to someone else, be sure to take a few seconds to easily post a quick positive review. As an author, your positive feedback is desperately needed. Your highly valuable five star reviews are like a river of golden joy flowing through a sunny forest of mighty trees and beautiful flowers! *To do your good deed in making the world a better place by helping others with your valuable insight, just leave a nice review.*

Thanks and Best of Luck

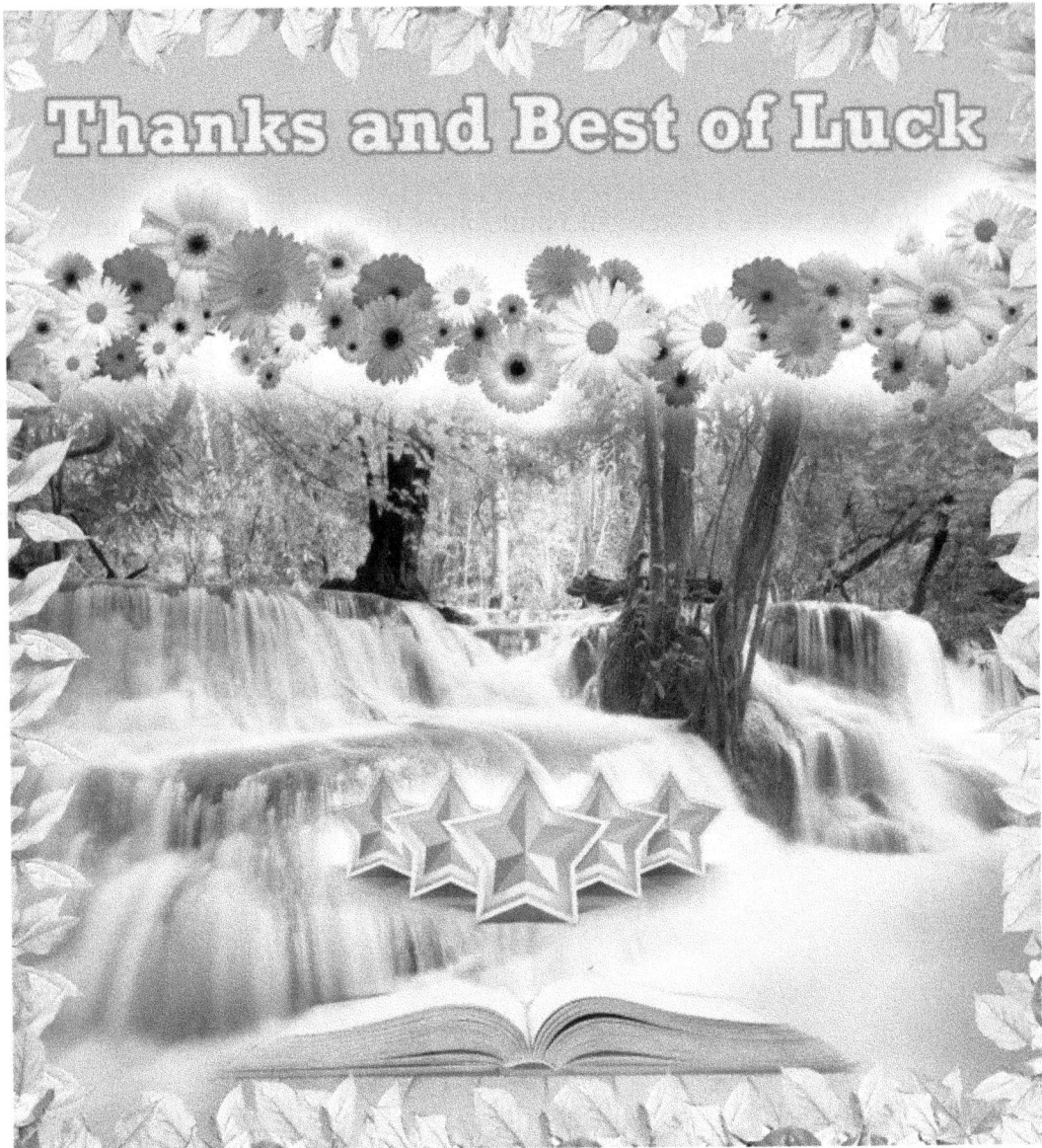

My Other Books and Audio Books
www.AcesEbooks.com

Health Books

ULTIMATE HEALTH SECRETS
HEALTH

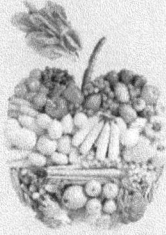

Strategies For Dieting, Eating Healthy, Exercising,
Losing Weight, The Mediterranean Diet,
Strength Training, And All About Vitamins,
Minerals, And Supplements

Ace McCloud

ENERGY
ULTIMATE ENERGY

Discover How To Increase
Your Energy Levels
Using The Best All Natural
Foods, Supplements
And Strategies For A Life
Full Of Abundant Energy

Ace McCloud

RECIPE BOOK

The Best Food Recipes
That Are Delicious, Healthy,
Great For Energy And Easy To Make

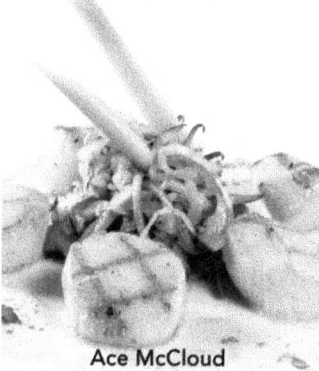

Ace McCloud

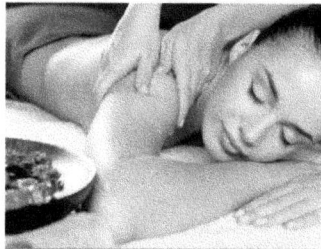

MASSAGE THERAPY

TRIGGER POINT THERAPY
ACUPRESSURE THERAPY
Learn The Best Techniques For
Optimum Pain Relief And Relaxation

Ace McCloud

LOSE WEIGHT

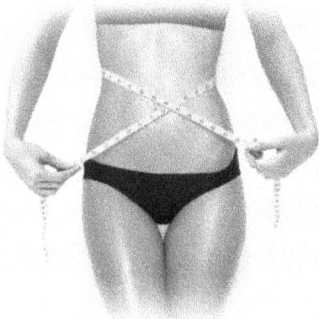

THE TOP 100 BEST WAYS
TO LOSE WEIGHT QUICKLY AND HEALTHILY

Ace McCloud

FATIGUE
OVERCOME CHRONIC FATIGUE

Discover How To Energize
Your Body & Mind So
That You Can Bring
The Energy & Passion
Back Into Your Life

Ace McCloud

Peak Performance Books

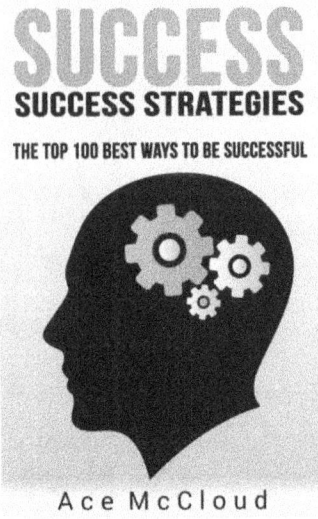

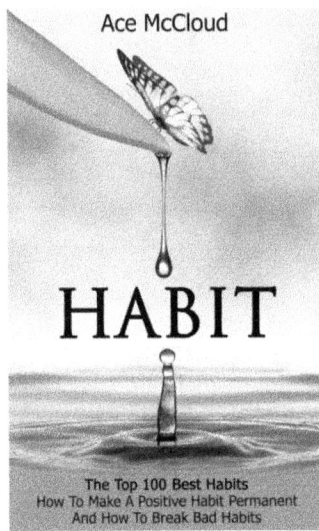

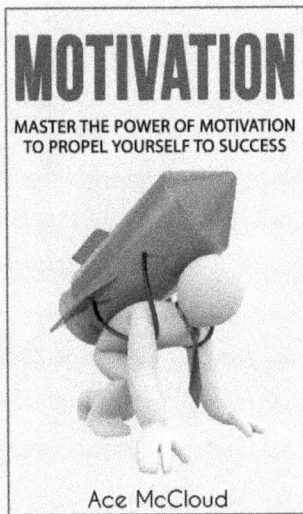

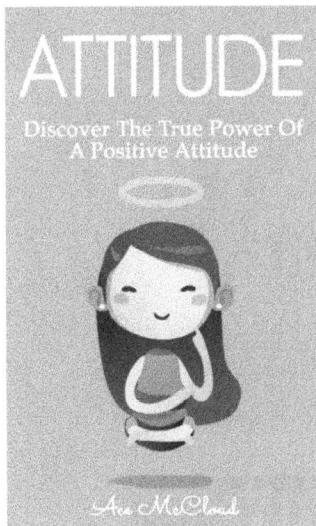

SUCCESS
SUCCESS STRATEGIES
THE TOP 100 BEST WAYS TO BE SUCCESSFUL

A c e   M c C l o u d

Ace McCloud

HABIT

The Top 100 Best Habits
How To Make A Positive Habit Permanent
And How To Break Bad Habits

MOTIVATION
MASTER THE POWER OF MOTIVATION
TO PROPEL YOURSELF TO SUCCESS

Ace McCloud

ATTITUDE
Discover The True Power Of
A Positive Attitude

Ace McCloud

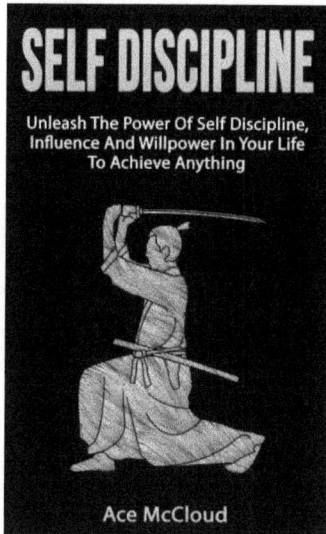

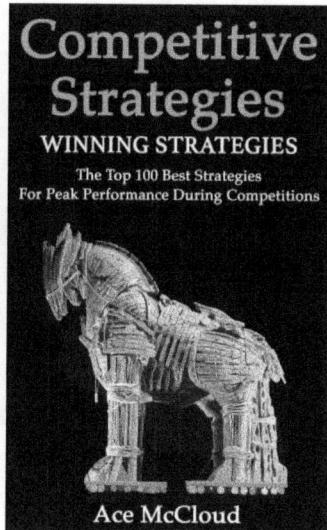

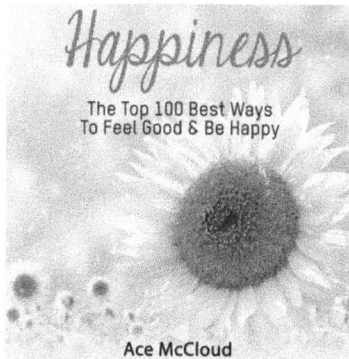

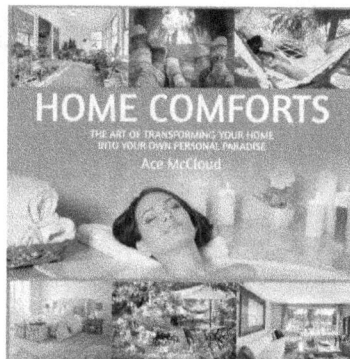

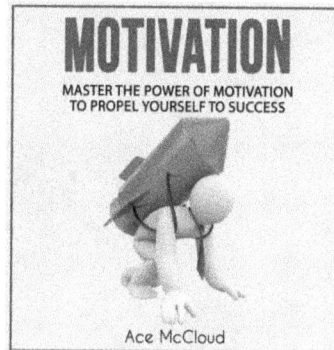

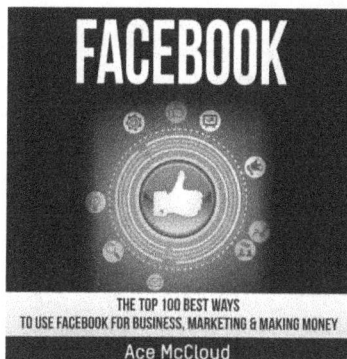

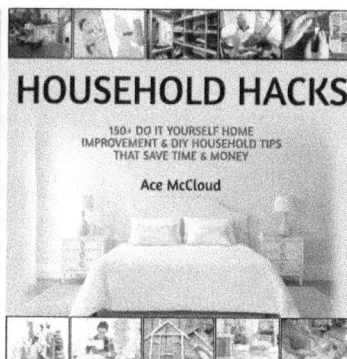

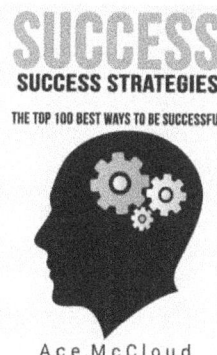

Check out my website at: www.AcesEbooks.com for a complete list of all of my books and high quality audio books. I enjoy bringing you the best knowledge in the world and wish you the best in using this information to make your journey through life better and more enjoyable! **Best of luck to you!**